THE GIFT

of

PAIN

THE GIFT

of

PAIN

Frederick W. Marks

EMMAUS
ROAD
PUBLISHING

Steubenville, Ohio
A Division of Catholics United for the Faith
www.emmausroad.org

Emmaus Road Publishing
827 North Fourth Street
Steubenville, Ohio 43952

Library of Congress Control Number: 2011945596
ISBN: 9781937155322

Cover design and layout by Theresa Westling

To my wife, Sylvia, who, along with my parents,
has taught me how to smile through pain.
And to my daughter, Mary Anne,
who has shown me how to embrace it.

TABLE OF CONTENTS

❖ ❖ ❖ ❖ ❖ ❖

INTRODUCTION

❖ ❖ ❖ ❖ ❖ ❖

Sweet are the uses of adversity.
—WILLIAM SHAKESPEARE

INTRODUCTION

❖ ❖ ❖ ❖ ❖ ❖

It is my hope that the following meditations on pain and suffering will be helpful to people of all faiths or none at all. At the same time, I firmly believe that nothing is more useful than religion in coming to terms with life's trials. Nothing is more uplifting; nothing is more profound. Jewish rabbis have said that tears are to the soul what soap is to the body. During the 700s, Habib al-Ajami, one of the Sufi saints of Islam, taught that suffering was a precious prize. Church of England apologist C. S. Lewis wrote that "God whispers to us in our pleasures, speaks in our conscience, but shouts in our pains."[1]

Catholicism in particular is noted for the breadth and depth of its writings on the subject of pain. Many of its greatest saints have actually prayed for it, and down through the years, its foremost leaders set an example of joyful renunciation in the way they embraced poverty, chastity, and obedience. When St. Benedict was tormented by temptations of the flesh, he threw himself, half naked, into a bed of thistles and thorns. It left him bleeding from head to toe, but never again was he tempted in the same way.

One might add that monks like Benedict were not the only ones who made use of pain. A large number of Catholic laymen and laywomen have done violence to their bodies for the sake of a higher good. Thomas More, Lord Chancellor of England under Henry VIII, wore a hair shirt until it bloodied him, even as he used a scourge on his back. Parenthetically, he was also the jolliest of souls and best of friends. Catherine of Siena (1347–80) ate almost nothing between the ages of six and twelve in order to enter into closer union with Christ. Yet she too was popular, indeed the most cheerful member of her family. Like More, she was brilliant and, like More, she scourged herself. Risking her life to relieve victims of the plague, sleeping for a mere half-hour at night, and subsisting for fifty-five days on the Eucharist alone, she was not only contagiously merry but charismatic enough to exert more influence on princes and potentates than any other person of her time.

I am trying to make the point that pain, in the eyes of the saint, is not something to be feared or

4

avoided. Rather, it is a tool that with proper use can bring us closer to God. When St. Andrew beheld the instrument of his crucifixion, he wept for joy at the thought of literally taking up his cross and following Christ. St. Rita of Cascia asked the Lord to let her feel the tip of a thorn so that she might share in the pain of Calvary, and the favor was granted. She developed a suppurating sore on her forehead that never went away. St. Rose of Lima, a woman of exquisite kindness, is worth quoting:

> If only mortals would learn how great it is to possess divine grace . . . they would devote all their care and concern to winning for themselves pains and afflictions. All men throughout the world would seek trouble, infirmities and torments, instead of good fortune, in order to attain the unfathomable treasure of grace. This is the reward and the final gain of patience. No one would complain about his cross or about troubles that may happen to him, if he would come to know the scales on which they are weighed when they are distributed to men.[2]

Spiritual athletes, like their counterparts in the Olympic arena, are people of courage. Like the runner who pushes himself until he drops, they go all out for God, and since they see Divine Providence as governing all, nothing ever appears accidental to them. Such things as "luck" and "fortune," which most of us take for granted, do not exist for the saint because he believes in a personal God who is all-knowing, all-powerful, and all-loving.

One doesn't have to be religious to feel comfortable with pain or to see the good that can come from it. But if suffering is to have meaning in a larger philosophical sense, and if we are to probe the nature of evil, we must turn to theology. Skeptics wince at the suggestion that cancer and natural disasters are gifts from above. How, they wonder, can God allow thousands upon thousands to be swept away from family and friends by tsunamis and earthquakes? How can the Father of Fathers permit a girl of twelve to die of leukemia before the eyes of parents who are down on their knees in prayer? How is it possible for one whom we call "all-good," "all-powerful," and "all-loving" to tolerate rape and genocide? How can God Almighty fashion creatures who are prone to such maniacal behavior?

Christianity and Judaism teach that murder, adultery, and other moral evils come not from God but from man, who, by virtue of the awesome gift of free will, can thwart the designs of Omnipotence. As for lesser forms of evil such as appendicitis and floods, the Book of Genesis traces their origin to original sin, and they are presented as God's remedy for human pride. Have you ever wondered what we would be like as human beings if it were it not for pain, suffering, and fear of death? On occasion, the saints themselves could be crusty and irascible. Paul, who had to live with some kind of "thorn in the flesh," saw his affliction as a gift to prevent him from becoming too elated (2 Cor. 12:7), and, as an agent of the Lord, he was perfectly willing to punish men *physically* to bring them to their senses *spiritually* (Acts 13:11; 1 Cor. 5:5). From his own experience on the road to Damascus—three days of blindness— he could vouch for the power of physical disability because it was this that led to his conversion.

Christian theologians may not be able to explain the motivation behind creation, but they do know the purpose of man, which is to know God, love Him, and serve Him in this world and to be happy with Him forever in the next. Knowing where we came from and where we are headed helps us reach our final destination, and religion assures us, secondly, that God will not send us more trouble than we can handle or allow the devil to tempt us beyond our power to resist (1 Cor. 10:13). Needless to say, this allows us to see temptation for what it is: namely, an invitation to grow in virtue.

Believers have the further advantage of being able to look forward to a glorious life in heaven provided they do their part. Pain is temporary and death is rebirth in the eyes of those who view life as a growing up process. Consider the analogous situation of a baby in pain. The child's problem could be gastrointestinal, or it could be teething. Whatever it is, the parents are not unduly alarmed because they anticipate a bright future for their offspring. And so it is with us. If we place our trust in God, we too can ride out life's difficulties knowing that, down the line, we have a bright future.

Still another consolation afforded by religion is derived from the many examples it sets before us of God meting out punishment to His most highly favored sons and daughters. With this in mind, we are less likely to interpret suffering as a sign of cosmic disfavor. The Book of Proverbs says that "the Lord reproves him whom he loves" (3:12). This is repeated in the Letter to the Hebrews (12:6), and we know that Jesus, along with His Blessed Mother, suffered the worst kind of cruelty and injustice.

Going a step further, the Christian is empowered to view pain as something that can be "offered up" for a share in Jesus' redemptive sacrifice on Calvary, and from this standpoint it is more of an asset than a liability. This point is clearly made by Peter (1 Pet. 4:13), as well as by Paul, who wrote that, "I rejoice in my sufferings for your sake, and in my flesh I complete what is lacking in Christ's afflictions for the sake of his body, that is, the church" (Col. 1:24).

I will close with two final references to ways in which belief in a personal God can give us the strength we need to bear up under pain. Most

Christians believe in purgatory, and along with it goes the assurance that whatever suffering we endure in this world will hasten our entrance to heaven after we die. Secondly, while there is no totally satisfying answer to the problem of why good men suffer, God is great and, if He is as great as we believe Him to be, mankind can no more fathom His grand design than a month-old baby can see the need to save for college. "My thoughts are not your thoughts, neither are your ways my ways, says the Lord" (Is. 55:8).

MEDITATION 1

◆ ◆ ◆ ◆ ◆ ◆

MARY THE MODEL

MARY THE MODEL

* * * * * *

Mel Gibson's film *The Passion of the Christ* created a sensation. Box office receipts soared, exceeding all expectations, and one of the questions still being asked is why? The film is brilliant from an artistic standpoint, and it also received a great deal of advance publicity due to its controversial nature, but beyond such factors lies something totally unique.

At a certain point in time, someone of inestimable stature chose to lay down his life in atonement for the sins of mankind. Such a thing had never been done before. It has never been done since. Jesus' action was at once so singular and so compelling that it should tell us something about Gibson's success. Any serious discussion of *The Passion* must come to grips with the meaning of suffering. Why did Christ suffer? Why do we suffer? What do we know about the results of pain? What does it mean to suffer as a Christian?

St. Thérèse of Lisieux wrote that suffering is "the best gift" God can give us, adding that "He gives it only to his chosen friends."[3]

She actually prayed for it, as St. Dominic and others had done. But her saying is not an easy one given our deep-seated instinct for self-preservation. We learn from childhood how to relieve every imaginable type of pain. Aspirin is a household word, and we head for the dentist when we have a toothache.

In a sense, we are quite right. Our bodies are temples of the Holy Spirit, and without health we couldn't put bread on the table or carry on a normal apostolate. Did Paul of Tarsus not ask God to remove the "thorn" in his flesh? Surely we offer similar prayers. The only difference is that we may be less philosophical than the man from Tarsus when God declines to give us what we want. Like Thérèse, Paul realized that suffering borne with faith can work to great advantage. "Power," he wrote, "is made perfect in weakness" (2 Cor. 12:9 NAB).

It is important to remember, when we encounter discomfort of any kind, that God is in charge. He will never send us anything not in our long-term best interest. Even atheists will allow that certain kinds of pain can be useful. Appendicitis, if not attended to immediately, is potentially fatal. When we feel a stabbing sensation on the right side of our abdomen, we are grateful for the warning. In the same way, fatigue produces soreness, which in turn signals the need for rest.

Most problems with pain stem from a lack of faith. We don't know, for example, when awakened in the middle of the night by a bad stomach upset, that the pain will soon subside and that it will never mount beyond our level of tolerance. Nine times out of ten, it is the uncertainty that hurts the most. And this is where prayer comes in. When we go to God for help, we can be sure (a) that He is listening and (b) that, though He may put us to the test, we will emerge from the ordeal stronger, happier, and humbler.

Some pain is self-imposed. During Lent we mortify ourselves. Fasting may cause our system to rebel, our tummy may rumble, we may experience weakness, headache, or coldness in the hands. Still, we are more fit. Not only are we better able to resist temptation, we are also leaner, more energetic, less susceptible to colds, and more alert. American Indian braves on the frontier used to fast before going on the warpath, and they were fierce. We, too, aim to be in topnotch physical condition. But for the Christian, fasting is mainly about solidarity with the Lord, testing one's willpower, and having a share in Jesus' sacrifice on Calvary.

Once we appreciate Lent's many benefits, the discipline appears less onerous. I remember how my daughter cried the first time I applied alcohol to a scraped knee. Later, after I explained the need to guard against infection, she took it matter-of-factly; she would even ask for it on occasion. I would then tell her with a twinkle in my eye that once one begins to associate pain with well-being, one is well along the path to maturity.

Mary illustrates to perfection the Christian concept of suffering. She is God's most highly favored daughter; yet never was a woman more heavily burdened. Beginning with the awkwardness during her betrothal to Joseph following the visit of the angel Gabriel, and ending with the persecution of her Son and His followers, she traversed miles and miles of sorrow.

As an expectant mother she could not find room at the inn. Nursing an infant she was driven into exile. How chagrined she must have been, in addition, to hear the story of the Innocents, knowing that if it hadn't been for the Nativity, none of Bethlehem's aggrieved would ever have felt the trauma of loss. The disappearance of her twelve-year-old Son for three days in the temple was but the prelude to another three-day agony. And then came the loss of her faithful spouse. It was under the pall of widowhood that she had to sustain the crushing blows that fell on Holy Thursday and Good Friday. Her third separation from Jesus occurred only forty days later, and this was followed by the execution of Stephen and James, son of Zebedee, who must have been among her nearest and dearest.

Finally, our Lady's life ended as it began, in total obscurity. Few, if any, of the movers and shakers of first century Rome had ever heard of her. Yet she was supremely powerful. Her influence exceeds that of all other women put together, in part because of the way she suffered. No one familiar with her plight can ever indulge in self-pity, react bitterly to discrimination, or lose hope in the providence of an all-loving Savior.

We thank God that Mary is our mother, given to each and every one of us by Our Lord on the Cross when He gave her to John (Jn. 19:26–27). Serenely self-effacing yet absolutely sure of herself, she is the patron of all who suffer, the queen of martyrs. We can go to her for help, confident that she will never turn away her face. But we must expect her to say to us what she said to the wedding attendants at Cana: "Do whatever he tells you" (Jn. 2:5 NAB). And we must expect further that her Son will tell us what He told the woman caught in adultery: "Go, and do not sin again" (Jn. 8: 11). God, the best of all parents, dispenses tough love.

MEDITATION 2

❖ ❖ ❖ ❖ ❖ ❖

APPEARANCE AND REALITY

APPEARANCE AND REALITY

❖ ❖ ❖ ❖ ❖ ❖

When the World Trade Center collapsed in a cloud of dust on 9/11/01, broadcasters focused on the wreckage. Faith-based newspapers, on the other hand, while not ignoring the devastation, called attention to a gigantic wrought-iron cross fashioned from free-falling girders, as if by the hand of God.

The secular media continues to concentrate on the wanton cruelty of a calculated assault on innocent life while we, in our Christian capacity, prefer to emphasize the good that has come of it—the heroism of the rescue teams, the return of millions to God, and the revival of patriotism. As people fed on the Bread of Angels, we draw inspiration from the words of Ecclesiastes: "Sorrow is better than laughter; because when the face is sad, the heart grows wiser." (7:3 NAB).

Benjamin Franklin, inventor of the lightning rod, regarded crippling diseases as a God-given opportunity to render service to his brothers and sisters in Christ. And how true. When Cardinal Egan celebrated Mass for Persons with Disabilities several years ago in St. Patrick's Cathedral, he told the folks on crutches, "I like to call you the enabling community because you enable us to give you a hand and do the work of the Lord." Volunteer efforts in response to the ghastly events of 9/11 were positively incredible. Among other things, churches benefited from the sale of patriotic pins handcrafted by enterprising parishioners.

Yes, there was death and destruction. But as Christians we believe there is nothing in life that cannot work to our advantage. Thus, there is no such thing as "premature death." Under the lens of faith, Providence replaces Lady Luck, and the only death that is premature is suicide. There is no such thing, moreover, as a "ripe old age." Every age is ripe when one is called home by God.

There is a tale about two women, each of whom had to bear up under the erratic behavior of an alcoholic husband. Each had a son and each at times felt terribly alone. Yet one of the boys would grow up to be president of the United States while the other would become America's poet laureate. Their names: Ronald Reagan and Robert Frost.

There was also a boy of nine who contracted diphtheria. So paralyzed were his arms and legs that he had to move about in a wheelchair. Later, his family lost its savings and he lacked the wherewithal to attend college. None of this seemed very promising. Nevertheless, the boy's name has since been indelibly stamped on the mind of everyone who knows American history: Harry Truman.

Let us suppose that, at the time of young Harry's crippling illness, his parents had been visited by an angel and told that their son was destined to occupy the nation's highest office. Assuming they took the angel at his word, this would have made all the difference.

And have we not received similar assurances? Did Jesus not promise us that we can outshine any president, prime minister, or lottery winner? Did He not pledge paradise to anyone serious about being a disciple? "Eye has not seen, nor ear heard, nor has it entered into the heart of man what things God has prepared for those who love him" (1 Cor. 2:9 CE).

Suffering, to be sure, is not easy. If it were, it would not be called "suffering." Life is fraught with difficulty. A commencement speaker, Thurgood Marshall, once told an audience of graduating seniors at the University of Michigan, "The world is waiting for you with open arms—and a club in each hand." Just so. We are put to the test. Yet, it is by this very testing that we are saved.

Those who suffer are spiritually better off than those who don't. But this is a fact that may not always be clear. When St. Paul wrote that women are saved by childbearing (1 Tim. 2:15), he assumed a degree of sophistication rare in any age. Most adults remain on a third-grade level when it comes to religious instruction. Tell almost any child about the value of homework and what does one get? A blank stare. Youngsters cannot see the forest for the trees, and such is the case when the average reader meets up with St. Paul.

When Our Lord said, "My yoke is easy, and my burden is light" (Mt. 11:30), He was not offering a life of ease, but rather ease of life for those willing to accept a share in His suffering. He came to proclaim the value of pain as a means of gaining eternal life. The Christian will not escape hardship and toil, much less illness and death. But, as we have already mentioned, he is strong to the degree that he can put such things to work by offering them up— hour by hour, day by day. We know this because Jesus showed us the way. He was not coerced; He accepted a cruel death in order to affirm the value of something the world holds in contempt.

Among the many advantages afforded by daily Bible reading is the opportunity to meet so many great men and women who dealt effectively with pain. All of God's prophets without exception faced opposition. Moses had to cope with widespread grumbling and rebellion, even treachery within his own family. Jeremiah, for his part, was imprisoned and tortured. Tradition tells us that Isaiah was sawed in two. And who has not heard of Job, who ran the gamut: financial ruin, devastating illness, and the loss of his entire family? Yet Job's patience is proverbial, and neither Moses nor Jeremiah nor Isaiah ever pointed the finger at God. None of them ever asked, "Why me?" Similarly in the case of the twelve apostles, ten of whom were blessed with martyrdom. Asked to pay the ultimate price, they paid it—and with joy. Peter had only one concern at the moment of execution. Loath to steal the Lord's glory, he begged to be crucified upside down.

There are times when God may act out of wrath. On occasion He will strike a sinner dead. But this never happens without an opportunity for repentance. Difficulties—the lot of every man—serve as so many wake-up calls. In this sense, famine and flood, along with pestilence and war, may be as useful to one's soul as peace and prosperity. When God sent Jewish armies into Canaan on a mission of extermination, it was owing to blatant immorality, and there had been ample time for a change of heart (Wis. 12). On the other hand, when He allowed Satan to strike at Job, He sought to make a man already rich in virtue richer still. In both cases, salvation was the aim.

When a true hero prostrates himself before the Lord in time of distress, his faith may waver, but it does not fail. He will receive sufficient grace to go on, and if he stays the course, he will fulfill his potential as a child of God.

Consider the example of Ludwig van Beethoven. As a concert pianist and musical composer, he knew no peer, but growing up he was subject to the demands of a heavy-drinking, dictatorial father. As an adult, he suffered disappointment in love, not to mention dozens of relocations and the ultimate tragedy for any musician: loss of hearing. None of the remedies prescribed by doctors for his disability proved of any avail, and the onset of deafness tempted him sorely to take his own life. Fortunately, faith enabled him to override frustration, and by persevering in his work, he reaped a harvest that was truly magnificent. Even today, his "Ode to Joy," which he never heard, lifts the hearts of millions.

Born, raised, and buried in the Catholic Church, Beethoven edged his desk with tributes to the power and glory of God, all of them neatly written out in his own hand, and he cared deeply about morality. "Recommend to your children virtue," he advised, since "that alone can make them happy, not gold." His one-time music teacher and lifelong idol, Joseph Haydn, father of classical music and originator of the symphony, often turned to the Rosary as a source of inspiration. One wonders if "Papa" Haydn did not bequeath to his protégé more than merely sound judgment in matters of musical composition.

MEDITATION 3

◆ ◆ ◆ ◆ ◆

PAIN AS A SHARPENER

PAIN AS A SHARPENER

❖ ❖ ❖ ❖ ❖ ❖

There is a saying that when the going gets tough, the tough get going. Juliette Low, founder of the Girl Scouts, is a case in point. On her wedding day, a grain of rice thrown on the bridal party lodged in her ear. Doctors tried to remove it, but in the process they pierced her eardrum, making her hard-of-hearing for life. It was a harbinger of things to come. Not only did her husband turn out to be a philanderer, he also left his entire fortune to his mistress. Juliette could have fallen to pieces; instead, she found a new channel for her love and spent herself for a worthwhile cause.

Another girl was barely six when her father and mother parted company. The stigma attached to divorce, combined with poverty, forced her family to move time and again. In spite of such obstacles—or perhaps on account of them—the girl grew up to be spiritually robust and eventually entered a convent. Some years later, she was severely injured when a heavy-duty scrubbing machine spun out of control. She managed to get back on her feet again, but the pain in her legs and back was so severe that it forced her to wear braces. The name of this remarkable woman, who went on to found a monastery in the South along with a Catholic media ministry that has inspired millions, is Mother Angelica.

There was also a boy from Kansas who was quite athletic. But on one occasion, while running, he fell and scraped his leg. Infection set in and he lapsed into delirium. Physicians, including specialists summoned from afar, feared for his life. His parents, forced to choose between amputation and grave risk of death, turned to prayer and simply commended their son to God.

The young man kept his leg. What's more, in spite of losing a full year of school, he was admitted to the United States Military Academy. Ironically, he suffered further leg injuries at West Point, forcing him to quit the football team and abandon his dream of becoming a cavalry officer. As head of a tank school in Pennsylvania during World War I, he couldn't obtain a single tank from Uncle Sam—only a few from France. And none of the tank officers who trained under him ever saw action on the front. As if this were not enough, his wife turned to drink, and things went from bad to worse. Yet the fear of God instilled in him during his childhood years in Abilene saw him through to a remarkable finish. His name: Dwight D. Eisenhower.

There will always be some who use suffering as an excuse to justify unbelief. As we have already observed, they want to know why God allows pain to torment good people if He himself is all-good and all-powerful. The question cuts deep and there is really no answer for those bent on skepticism. As Christians, though, we find a definitive answer in Jesus, who, in order to save the world, suffered the worst pain the world has ever been able to inflict. God could have accomplished His purpose any way He wanted. But He used suffering as an instrument to show us the way.

In the Old Testament, the immolation of the lamb was a sign of salvation. In the New Covenant, Jesus, of course, is the Lamb of salvation. And in both cases, the principle is the same. As St. Paul wrote, "Without the shedding of blood there is no forgiveness of sins" (Heb. 9:22). Perhaps this is why the deaf, when they refer to Our Lord in sign language, point to the palms of their hands and to imaginary nail prints of crucifixion. Such marks are of the essence, for our religion was born in pain. We are not surprised to find that "into every life a drop of rain must fall" and no one has to tell us that without rainfall there would be no crops.

Along with Christ's example, there are innumerable case studies indicating that pain can lead to greatness. Babe Ruth, the home-run king, struck out 1,300 times before he reached the hall of fame, and Abraham Lincoln lost more elections than he won. History suggests further that suffering is the gateway to creativity. It is highly doubtful that Charles Dickens would have written *David Copperfield* or *Oliver Twist* had he been financially secure. And the same may be said of others. Walter Scott, like Dickens, was forced by the pinch of penury to harness his literary talent. Both men were indebted to debt.

Next in importance to indebtedness as a catalyst for greatness comes disability. In the case of Thomas Edison, Alexander Graham Bell, and S. F. B. Morse, it could well be argued that without the deafness that plagued members of the families of all three men and vigorous efforts on the part of each to overcome its effects, none of them would have made their mark. The light bulb, the phonograph, and Morse Code are all products of persistent efforts to deal with a handicap.

Third and fourth on our list as agents of progress are melancholy and death—once again, entirely unlikely from a strictly secular point of view. How many of us are aware that the most famous of all waltzes and the most beloved of all marches owe their existence to one or another form of sadness? Johann Strauss conceived *The Blue Danube* while meditating on a poem about a woman "rich in sadness," while John Philip Sousa was mourning the death of a close friend and business associate when he composed his *Stars and Stripes Forever*.

And one can go further. When the author of *Black Beauty* first put pen to paper, her doctor had given her just eighteen months to live. Then there is Harvard's Widener Library, one of academia's greatest book repositories, built because Mr. and Mrs. Widener, the parents of a man drowned in the tragic sinking of the *Lusitania* in 1915, wanted to commemorate their son's life and untimely death at sea by establishing a fund for the promotion of scholarship.

Occasionally, one comes across a saga in which almost all of the above elements come into play. Such is the case with Theodore Roosevelt. TR would never have become a judo expert and boxing champion, much less McKinley's successor in the White House, had it not been for asthma. As a child, he hovered at death's door during chronic fits of wheezing. But he would not admit defeat and what emerged from his decades-long battle for fitness was an outstanding physique, along with sterling character. When a would-be assassin fired point-blank at him in 1912 during his "Bull Moose" campaign, the bullet met three objects along its path: a speech manuscript, an eyeglass case, and a powerful set of upper-body muscles developed during Roosevelt's childhood fight for survival. The Rough Rider, about to deliver a speech, paid little heed to the bullet. Indeed, he insisted on delivering the entire text of his address with a slug buried deep in his chest!

This first Roosevelt, not to be confused with distant cousin Franklin (FDR), was one of the last of the Renaissance men: big game hunter, cowboy, soldier, police commissioner, governor, author of dozens of books, historian, natural scientist, and, not least of all, family man. And just as his career was multifaceted, so, too, was his suffering.

As a freshman legislator in New York's State Assembly, he received word that things were sadly amiss at home. Boarding the first train to Manhattan, he proceeded to lose through death the two most important women in his life, his wife and mother, within a matter of hours. Such pain, excruciating for a man of Roosevelt's affectionate nature, might have caused him to fall prey to self-pity. But not TR, who retreated to the Dakota Badlands, got back on his feet, and forged full steam ahead.

Earlier, during his years at Harvard, he had taught Sunday school and to the end of his life he would stress the importance of weekly church attendance. Thus, sustained by religious faith during the darkest days of his life, he was able to rise meteorically to the governorship of New York and from there to the Oval Office, from whence he inaugurated the Square Deal, instituted the National Park System, and won the Nobel Peace Prize.

Around the time TR was fending off asthma attacks, a young Italian was reeling under similar blows. Within the space of three years, he lost his entire family—a wife and two sons—and like his American counterpart, he refused to admit defeat. As an altar boy, he had nearly fainted with rapture when he first heard the sound of the organ at his local church. Now, supremely challenged, he nursed a talent for musical composition and flung himself headlong into what he knew best. Fusing childlike faith in God with incandescent zeal, he not only survived but surpassed himself by turning out scores such as *Rigoletto, II Trovatore,* and *Aida.* The world was richer for his perseverance, and this same Giuseppe Verdi closed out his career with a successful foray into national politics.

Pain, when it rubs against character, acts as a sharpener. Would Verdi or the first Roosevelt have joined the ranks of the immortals without being hammered nearly to death on the anvil of "misfortune"? They might have done well. But would they have achieved wonders? Fyodor Dostoevsky might have been a good man had he not been sentenced to hard labor in a Siberian prison camp. But years of toil combined with meditation on the Bible, the only book allowed in his cell, had a powerful effect. This, in addition to a dramatic eleventh-hour stay of execution that saved his life (a firing squad actually stood at the ready) converted him to Christianity, and from that moment on, he soared. *Crime and Punishment* and *The Brothers Karamazov* were only a matter of time.

Not many years ago, a Peruvian hostage crisis received broad coverage in the press. Shining Path guerrillas, after seizing the Japanese embassy in Lima, held dignitaries hostage for weeks. While radical demands were negotiated, lives hung in the balance. Eventually, through the mediation of Church authorities, a logjam was broken and the captives were freed. From a purely human standpoint, the episode was terrifying. But out of it came a corps of heroes—people determined to change their lives and, in particular, to dedicate themselves to their families as never before. God is in charge, and an act of terrorism, like any other act, is the raw material from which saints are made.

Some time ago, I myself reached a spiritual plateau after being hijacked on a trans-Atlantic flight by Palestinian gunmen. For a brief period following this extremely close brush with death, I experienced a heightened appreciation for the gift of life, along with an increased sensitivity to the needs of others. But then it was back to normal. My sainthood lasted approximately six weeks! I will say this, however: I caught a glimpse of the value of pain.

MEDITATION 4

◆ ◆ ◆ ◆ ◆ ◆

GREAT DISAPPOINTMENTS

GREAT DISAPPOINTMENTS

❖ ❖ ❖ ❖ ❖ ❖

Just as germs in diluted form may be used to inoculate against illness, so too may God use bitterness as a sweetening agent. An attack by poisonous snakes brought grumbling Israelites to their senses under Moses, and David, having added murder to adultery, realized the enormity of his offense when his first-born son died in infancy. Thomas à Becket, England's great martyr-saint, was wild as a lad. But one day he nearly drowned and, as he was about to go under, he vowed that if his life was spared he would dedicate what remained of it to the Lord. Along the same line, David Goldstein, an American apologist of the early 1900s, used to say that Jewish suffering over the centuries was God's way of calling his people home. And so it was.

The divine tug on the sleeve will often come in ways that seem quite natural. Evelyn Waugh, the British literary convert, became so depressed as an adolescent that he sought to take his life by wading into deep water. Before wading very far, however, he was stung by a jellyfish. In a split second, all thought of suicide vanished and a brilliant writing career opened up. St. Norbert, every bit as frivolous as Becket and Waugh, was struck by lightning. Miraculously, he survived, and his life changed completely. For Miguel de Cervantes, author of *Don Quixote*, it took three gunshot wounds in the Battle of Lepanto followed by captivity and the loss of a hand.

The afflictions suffered by children have been a major cause of parental awakening. Alexander Hamilton, Clare Boothe Luce, and Alec Guinness were greatly different in terms of career, but they had two interesting things in common. First, all three experienced religious conversion, two of them to Catholicism (Luce and Guinness). Luce served in the United States Congress and represented her country overseas, Guinness won world renown as a comic actor, and Hamilton rose from obscurity and parental neglect two centuries earlier to become America's first Secretary of the Treasury. The second bond linking our threesome is the fact that their spiritual rebirth came about as a direct result of tragedy in the family, tragedy specifically involving a child.

Hamilton's story is especially poignant. Not until his eldest son was killed in a duel defending his father's honor did the treasury secretary think seriously about the meaning of life. Crushed by the loss of his son and further stunned when the boy's lovely sister, Angelica, plunged from grief to insanity, he began studying the Bible and reading Christian apologetics. He led the family in prayer and grew visibly in both warmth and generosity. In 1804, Aaron Burr challenged him to a duel he felt honor-bound to accept. But on Christian principle, he resolved not to take his opponent's life, and the day before he was fatally wounded by Burr, he knelt with his twelve-year-old son and recited the Lord's Prayer, believing to the end that "the will of a merciful God must be good."

All of which causes one to ponder the meaning of success and failure. George Washington, who led men into battle seven times, was defeated seventy percent of the time. During the War for Independence, he spent nearly all of his time on the defensive. Yet he became the father of his country.

One is reminded of the Brontë sisters of Haworth, England, who traveled all the way to Brussels to learn how to run a school. But when they returned to England and mailed out a prospectus for the academy they hoped to found, no one answered. And so they turned to writing. Charlotte is best known as the author of *Jane Eyre*.

Then there is St. Benedict, the father of western monasticism, who was so unpopular with the monks who first served under his aegis that they tried to poison him.

The lives of the great are positively strewn with disappointment. John Bosco, founder of the Salesian Order, failed to found a seminary while Cardinal Newman tried in vain to bring out an updated English translation of the Bible; his hopes for a Catholic university were also dashed.

Still another on history's list of distinguished failures is Elizabeth Seton, founder of the parochial school system in the United States. She tried to obtain a cure for her dying husband, but it was not to be. Shortly after her conversion to Catholicism, and partially on account of it, she had to give up teaching. Her school closed, and owing to the social wrath kindled by the conversion of her sister-in-law, she could not even run a boarding house for motherless boys. Finally, she died wondering what kind of an impression she had made on her own children.

Such frustration, but one of the many faces of suffering, is closely related to another form of hardship known to all: namely, the hiding of one's future. Take the story of St. Anthony of Padua. He yearned from the bottom of his soul to evangelize the Muslims of North Africa, but malaria forced him to retreat. On his way home to native Portugal, a storm diverted his ship to Italy, and while there he was assigned menial chores in a monastery kitchen. There he stayed for a time, but as God would have it, one of the preachers eventually fell ill. Anthony was assigned to take his place in the pulpit, and the rest is history. He knew the entire Bible by heart and before long his fiery preaching was in demand the world over.

Like Anthony, Ignatius and Francis dreamed of becoming missionaries to Islam, but God had other plans. Ignatius' failure to realize his fondest hope forced the Jesuits to enter the field of teaching, and of course this has been their forte ever since. Father Flanagan, founder of Boy's Town in Nebraska, encountered similar reverses. Repeatedly, he had to drop out of the seminary on account of illness. Only after many false starts did he finally complete his coursework, overseas.

Why, one wonders, does it so often take sadness or death, danger or frustration, to put life in proper perspective? Illusion seems to be part and parcel of the human condition. Two millennia ago, Jesus chafed at stiffened necks and hardened hearts, eyes that did not see and ears that did not hear. Has anything changed? Unless we are shocked into a connection with the real world, we remain hopelessly mired in the mush of utopia. Why must certain types of parents experience a miscarriage before they learn respect for human life? According to one OB-GYN, who has testified to the power of failed pregnancy to produce determined foes of abortion, "it is only when we suffer that we can truly see and know ourselves."[4]

The fact is that there are few in any day or age who truly appreciate the gift of life. Almost always, we take it for granted. Likewise with those who suffer: they rarely appreciate the gift of pain. If those *in extremis* only knew that they could offer every hour of every day in atonement for sin—their own as well as that of others—how encouraged they would be! When Mary appeared to the children of Fatima in 1917 and asked if they were ready to accept all the suffering God might send them for the conversion of sinners, all three said yes, and all three suffered terribly. Jacinta and Francisco, who begged Mary to take them with her to heaven, perished in the flu epidemic of 1919–20. Lucia, for her part, survived for over eighty additional years to face cold indifference on the part of those who would continue to turn their back on the most thoroughly authenticated miracle of all time.

Closer to home, an American girl by the name of Donna Camilleri was born not long ago with Down Syndrome. There had been no history of such illness in the family and when her mother heard the news she cried her heart out. But Donna's birth proved to be a blessing, for it brought her brothers and sisters closer to God. Why, she typically wanted to know, did the family offer mealtime prayer only at Christmas and Easter? Why not at every meal? Her father, in appreciation of his "victim soul" daughter, remarked, "She is pure goodness and has changed everyone in the family for the better."[5]

MEDITATION 5

◆ ◆ ◆ ◆ ◆ ◆

THE GREAT TRANSFORMER

THE GREAT TRANSFORMER

❖ ❖ ❖ ❖ ❖ ❖

Many have heard about how a lowly thistle inspired the discovery of Velcro. Perhaps they know too about how an accidental spilling of sulfur and rubber onto a hot stove led to the process known as vulcanization. But how many have ever stopped to think about how God is constantly bringing good out of evil with the aid of his children? That Mary Magdalene should have wept copious tears at the feet of Jesus and embraced Him with such fervor must have been due in part to the fact that, with the help of Our Lord, she managed to lift such a heavy burden from her shoulders, rising from bedeviled beginnings to sainthood. As Jesus remarked to the Pharisees, "he who is forgiven little, loves little" (Lk. 7:47). Even the fall of Adam and Eve can be viewed as having worked to our advantage, for without it not one of us would have access to heaven. It is for this reason that original sin is sometimes referred to as "the fortunate fall."

Children's literature is full of the wonder of God's transforming power. When the tears of the *Velveteen Rabbit* fall to the ground, they produce a mysterious flower from which issues "the loveliest fairy in the whole world," and this fairy proceeds to set things straight. Wrongs are righted, happiness is restored. Beauty's tears, falling on the lifeless Beast, are again redemptive because they transform him into a handsome prince.

Poverty, too, has its flip side. People born on New York's Lower East Side during the Great Depression had little to their name. Yet later in life many of them cherished fond childhood memories. Not until they grew up did they realize that their families had been poor. They had just as much fun, if not more, than those born on Park Avenue, and for the simple reason that happiness comes from within. It doesn't depend on accidentals like wealth or place of birth. Many who are restless think that by relocating they will discover the magic that is missing in their lives. But chances are that if they are unhappy in Timbuktu they will be unhappy in New York. Conversely, if they are happy where they are and are forced to move, they will take their happiness with them.

Charles Dickens developed this point at some length in a number of works, including his beloved *Christmas Carol*, where the poorest characters turn out to be the happiest. Dickens was an astute analyst of human nature, and what he recorded is what he saw. Every day, individuals blessed with good health wear long faces. By the same token, we have all met handicapped individuals who radiate joy. Fr. Paul Marx, OSB, founder of Human Life International, once visited a facility for lepers run by the Missionaries of Charity. The residents were terribly disfigured, but he came away certain that he had never seen "a happier lot of men and women." Statistics tell us that there is a lower suicide rate among paraplegics than among the healthy, further that millionaires are more likely to take their lives than are paupers. Where there is faith, there is hope, and when people are good, they are happy. God is the great transformer.

Jesus' choice of the word "blessed" to describe the poor (Lk. 6:20) is significant, and St. James leaves no doubt that such blessing applies to those who are physically poor, as well as "poor in spirit." The same term is used by Our Lord to describe "those who mourn" (Mt. 5:4), and once again, a look at the record turns up suggestive glimmerings. Two of the most popular musical composers of all time, Wolfgang Amadeus Mozart and Ludwig van Beethoven, were raised by mothers who began life's journey in orphanages run by nuns. And to the names of gifted children brought up by orphaned women may be added the names of those who were themselves orphans, among them Ambrose, Copernicus, Magellan, and Ignatius. Catherine McAuley, who founded a religious order that opened more schools in English-speaking countries than any other, lost her father at the tender age of five and her mother thirteen years later.

The list of Americans who lost at least one of their parents in childhood reads like a "Who's Who in the USA." We have George Washington, Thomas Jefferson, Benjamin Franklin, Andrew Jackson, Abraham Lincoln, Robert E. Lee, Andrew Carnegie, John Jacob Astor, Mark Twain, Theodore Roosevelt, Louis Armstrong, Joe Louis, Franklin Roosevelt, and Jackie Robinson. Non-Americans in the same category include Confucius, Alexander the Great, Julius Caesar, Caesar Augustus, St. Jerome, St. Augustine, Dante, Michelangelo, Pascal, Caruso, and Solzhenitsyn.

A similar list could be compiled of great men and women who grew up in large families. To have a healthy complement of siblings is hardly a matter for mourning, but it can pose a problem. There is less space to go around, less parental attention, less money, and less peace and quiet. Hand-me-downs are the one thing found in abundance. Nonetheless, statistical evidence, once more, confirms the underlying truth of the Beatitudes. Individuals raised in families with ten or more youngsters include Thomas Jefferson, James Madison, Washington Irving, St. Ignatius, St. Rose of Lima, Joseph Haydn, Franz Schubert, John Philip Sousa, Arthur Conan Doyle, and Father Flanagan, the founder of Boy's Town.

If we were to extend the list to include persons with fifteen or more brothers and sisters, we could add Albrecht Dürer, the greatest woodcarver, sketcher, and engraver of all time, along with John Marshall, arguably the most distinguished of all Chief Justices of the U.S. Supreme Court. Also included are Ben Franklin, Harriet Beecher Stowe, and Enrico Caruso. Catherine of Siena, the greatest woman of the fourteenth century, and Thomas Aquinas, one of the Church's foremost philosophers, both grew up in families of twenty or more children. Surely St. Paul had it right when he observed that "the foolishness of God is wiser than men" (1 Cor. 1:25 CE).

Continuing to search history's storeroom for the meaning of the Beatitudes, one finds still another clue: Christianity has always been strongest in areas of the world that are the least prosperous. Since 1960, the number of vocations to the priesthood and religious life has soared in Africa and, to a lesser degree, Latin America and South Asia, while in the industrialized West it has fallen dramatically. Similarly, we know that prostitutes and publicans showed more interest in Jesus' teachings than people of the establishment (such as the Pharisees and Sadducees), also that St. Paul was more successful with the scapegraces of Corinth than he was with Athens' elite.

After Constantine built his new capital in the East, Byzantine culture and affluence carried the day. Yet it was in the West the Faith blossomed most fully. The East certainly produced its saints, men of the caliber of Basil and Chrysostom, but none of them have been as influential as Augustine or Jerome. The East also turned out great rulers, but none so great as Charlemagne, Stephen, and Otto. Nor should it be forgotten that Constantinople succumbed to the Arian heresy, whereas Rome clung steadfastly to orthodoxy. It is a simple fact that Christ's divinity was denied by *all* of the Eastern Sees at one time or another, but never by the pope. A thousand years later, the pattern ran true to form when Europe split in two over the Protestant Revolt. People were more faithful to tradition and to the Holy Father in southern areas, which remained Catholic, than in northern ones that claimed greater wealth. Blessed are the poor.

Consider, finally, the sites of the greatest miracles since the time of the Resurrection. Guadalupe in 1531 was marginal from an economic standpoint, while Mexico City was thriving. Three centuries later, Lourdes was struggling while Paris boomed. In 1917, Fatima was a backwater in comparison with Lisbon. Without exception, Christ has manifested

Himself most spectacularly in places where the people were poor and the Faith rich.

Power corrupts. One of the most telling facts of our own era is the speed with which Muslims, who come from less privileged countries, are beginning to overtake Christians in terms of sheer numbers. Mosques are going up everywhere and with burgeoning numbers comes increased political power. A mighty change is in the offing. Why? Because Muslims are cognizant of something that many Christians, especially in the industrialized West, seem to have forgotten: namely, every child is a gift from God. The women of Islam are risking pregnancy, and the men are opening their wallets in order to glorify their Creator. They may not possess the full truth, but what they possess they cherish. It is a sad commentary on contemporary Catholicism that when the Holy Father opposes UN-sponsored efforts to promote abortion, sterilization, and contraception, he finds more support among Muslims than among his own people.

What is happening today in the industrialized West is sadly reminiscent of what happened in Israel at the time of Elijah, Elisha, and Jesus. There were many Jewish widows, but none as deserving as a pagan woman of Zarephath (1 Kings 17:8–24). There were many Jewish lepers, but none as worthy of God's healing touch as Naaman the Syrian (2 Kings 5). There were many Jews with faith, but none with the faith of a Roman centurion (Mt. 8:5–13).

MEDITATION 6

◆ ◆ ◆ ◆ ◆ ◆

THE SNOWSTORM OF LIFE

THE SNOWSTORM OF LIFE

❖ ❖ ❖ ❖ ❖ ❖

A cheery fellow who lives next door to me will often remark on how lovely the weather is, and when someone replies, "I hear it's going to rain to-morrow," he shoots back, "True, but after the rain comes the sun!" When a curbstone philosopher tells him that health is the most important thing in life, his answer never varies: "Thank God for our health, but even more for the faith that sustains us through thick and thin and makes us happy in the hospital, as well as on the beach," or words to that effect.

This neighbor of mine sees a silver lining in every cloud, and perhaps he is overly optimistic. Some might call him a Pollyanna. One thing, though, is certain: He doesn't suffer, as naysayers do, from tunnel vision. A story is told of an old farmer whose only horse ran away. In sympathy, his fellow villagers said, "What misfortune you have!" In reply, the farmer said, "There is no misfortune, only blessings in disguise!" A few days later, his horse returned with a dozen wild horses following along! The villagers said, "What good fortune you have!" The farmer replied, "There is no good fortune, only God's will!" Shortly afterward, his only son was thrown from one of the wild horses and sprained his back. The villagers again cried, "What bad fortune you have!" Then, a few days later, his son was supposed to march into war but was excused because of his injury! The farmer declared, "If you trust in God, then there are only blessings or blessings in disguise!"

To many, the notion of pain as a gift sounds strange, if not bizarre. It is only natural to regard people as well-off when they have health and wealth, power and popularity. But, as we all know, what is natural is not always correct. Edwin Arlington Robinson, one of Theodore Roosevelt's favorite authors, wrote a short poem entitled "Richard Cory," which makes the point with a bang. Every time Cory, the central character, walks down the street he is envied for his good looks, imperial grace, intelligence, and riches. He has everything in life one could ask for *except pain*, and in the last line of Robinson's masterpiece, he puts "a bullet through his head." Success measured in worldly terms does not have to make one happy.

The flip side of the coin is that pain, in the sense of anguish or deprivation, need not make one sad. When I was eighteen, my father took me to Haiti, which, long before the tragedy of the recent earthquake, was the poorest country in the western hemisphere, and what I remember most vividly is all the smiling faces. People on the roads and in the marketplaces were poor by our standards, but never have I seen so many happy-looking souls.

Just as we find it hard to imagine joy in poverty, there are times when we miss the connection between suffering and goodness. Those who grew up in the years following World War II will recall that one of the more common expressions was "Good grief!" It is an oxymoron seldom heard nowadays, but it contains an important element of truth. The kindest and dearest people are generally those who have suffered the most. Conversely, those for whom things have gone well are apt to be on the proud side. In the family classic, *I Remember Mama*, one of the characters says that to suffer is "to have a little good in you," and G. K. Chesterton once observed that to be in hot water is a good thing because this is how one keeps clean. Suffering has been likened to a crucible, as well as a furnace, for refining precious metal. Jesus speaks of it as a form of baptism (Mk. 10:38), and there are places in the New Testament where it is compared to the process of pruning (e.g.,

Jn. 15:2). Just so. Like vines, shrubs, and trees, we all need an occasional trimming if we are to live up to our potential.

"It's an ill wind that blows no good," they say, and those who have flown in turbulent weather know what happens when one's plane gets shaken for any length of time by a wind that is literally "ill." There is much soul-searching aboard the aircraft, along with nail-biting, and when the rubber of the wheels finally touches the tarmac, the passengers breathe a sigh of relief. They relax, exchange pleasantries, and, through a shared experience, are brought closer together.

It is much the same in my hometown, New York, when a heavy snowstorm blows in. The snowflakes mount up over patches of ice, and people begin to slip and fall, especially the elderly. Traffic grinds to a halt. Cars are entombed and there is an immense amount of digging to be done. Still, it is precisely in the grip of a blizzard that people begin to converse, even the shyest and most reserved. Help is offered, equipment is shared, errands are run, and it doesn't even have to snow. All it takes is a sudden rise or fall in the temperature to tease out dimples and loosen tongues.

In some cases, it may take years to see the underside of suffering because people in the grip of an emergency are seldom reflective. During the Great Depression, the problems facing the nation were daunting. Men lost fortunes and some jumped from the tops of tall buildings. Yet out of widespread misery came a wonderful generosity of spirit. Halos appeared in unlikely places. Joy sprouted from despair. Pride broke down under the solvent of tribulation. Goodness had a field day.

The next worst thing to financial panic in worldly terms is time in prison. But even here, the results can be surprising. Alexander Solzhenitsyn's novella, *A Day in the Life of Ivan Denisovich*, features a prisoner who finds happiness in Siberia, and the story of Ivan is played out every day in the real world. Victor Frankel, in *Man's Search for Meaning*, tells of how faith sustained the inmates of German concentration camps during World War II, and one can cite numerous instances of incarceration bringing people to God. Guy Gruters, a Vietnam POW for five years, said that he had never been happier than when he found the Lord in prison and exchanged a nominal form of Catholicism for the real thing. It was on the anvil of torture and humiliation that he shook off false pride, along with temptations to suicide, and while he was being hammered, his wife and two youngsters remained faithful back in the States—so faithful, in fact, that after his release, she converted and bore him five more children!

Thus far, we have focused on the effect of hardship on those directly affected. But suffering, borne cheerfully, can influence a wide range of witnesses. Who can pass a blind man with a cane in his hand and a smile on his face without being ashamed of one's petty complaints? Such saints as Bernadette and Josemaría Escrivá profited enormously from the example of parents who faced financial ruin with Christian equanimity. J. R. R. Tolkien, the author of the best-selling *Lord of the Rings*, was similarly moved by his widowed mother's loyalty to the Catholic Faith at a time in her life when conversion from Protestantism left her without friends or family. In America, John D. Rockefeller, the industrial giant, never forgot the way his devout mother bore up under accusations of rape leveled at her absentee husband, who spent much of his time on the road.

Or take an incident that occurred on September 9, 2005, during the women's semifinals of the U.S. Open Tennis Championship. A French woman by the name of Mary Pierce, plagued for years with injuries, was playing a heavily favored Russian, and after several tough sets, she won. Asked on the aftermath of the game how she had managed to pull off an incredible upset, she replied, with tears welling up in her eyes, that she had thought of a friend who was ill and this gave her the power.

Those who suffer nobly can make conquests even on their deathbed. Saul, affected by the magnanimity with which Stephen, the first Christian martyr, gave up his spirit, became Paul; and Edith Stein, recently canonized, was so impressed with the joy, cheerfulness, and composure with which a Catholic friend of hers died that it put her on the road to conversion. Death itself can be uplifting. On news of the passing of Pope John Paul II, many came to confession who had not seen a priest in ages. When Chateaubriand, the great French author and statesman, returned to the Catholic fold after having been away for many years, he attributed it in large part to the deaths of his mother and one of his sisters. "I wept and I believed,"[6] he wrote. Or take the case of Don Juan, a real person who lived many years ago in the city of Seville. He was very wealthy, very generous, and very loose. But the mere sight of a funeral procession changed his life completely as he pondered the hollowness of vanity and transience of glory. *Sic gloria transit mundi.*

It is a truism that genius is 98% perspiration, and what is perspiration if not another word for pain? Nothing great is ever accomplished without it. No pain, no gain. It is only human to try to escape suffering, but the flight from what is part and parcel of the human condition can lead to alcoholism, promiscuity, and drug abuse. For some, it is simply the road to mediocrity. My mother used to read me *The Little Engine That Could,* about a steam locomotive trying to make its way up a steep grade with more heart than horsepower and, in the end, succeeding. I think she was trying to get across the idea that we are all little engines that must learn to live by gumption, faith, and perseverance.

The vast majority of first-time business enterprises fail, and if one studies the lives of the greats, whether they be engineering wizards or sports champions, one sees a single pattern: patience and long suffering in the face of adverse circumstances. Geniuses like Thomas Edison failed hundreds of times for every time they succeeded. What if Edison had given up during his initial experiments? What if Olympic track star Wilma Rudolph had been cowed into inactivity by her childhood braces? What if Tour de France winner Lance Armstrong had given in to cancer?

Walk in the footsteps of a saint and you will find a trail of tears. St. Patrick, who converted Ireland, and St. Vincent de Paul, who invented organized charity as we know it today, were both kidnapped by pirates. Both spent years in slavery. But far from languishing, they grew in holiness. Monsieur Vincent, as he is called in his native France, escaped his captors and was ordained to the priesthood. But no sooner was he launched on his career as a servant of God than he was falsely accused of stealing. Calumny hung over his reputation for what seemed an eternity until the real culprit finally confessed. He also faced the deadly plague, and later, as a royal official, he felt it his duty to disappoint influential members of the nobility by blocking the appointment of their unworthy sons and daughters to high posts in the Church. None of this was pretty, but though he didn't know it at the time, none of it would hold him back.

Here are a few more examples of saintly individuals who persisted in the face of opposition to what they believed to be the will of God. When Mother Teresa of Calcutta sought to build a shelter for the destitute in an affluent neighborhood, she received death threats, but she kept building. Mother Angelica, the founder of EWTN, the largest religious broadcasting station in the world, saw bullets whiz through the windows of her convent when she first moved to Birmingham, Alabama, but she too kept on going even after the shooting occurred a second time. Not everyone liked her. She used to say that she often felt like a porcupine at a balloon party! But she was not a quitter, and she attributed all of her accomplishments to "a foundation of pain."[7]

Then there is John Audubon, celebrated painter of wildlife, especially birds, who was tempted to throw away his brushes when rats attacked a box containing several hundred of his favorite canvasses, ruining the entire lot. Instead, he spent three years retouching, and when he couldn't find a publisher in the United States, he went to England where his collection, now world famous, was published as *Birds of North America.*

What if Joan of Arc had been less insistent in her quest to lead the armies of France? There was no red carpet laid out for her at the palace of the Dauphin! What if Christ's apostles, after being flogged for preaching in the Temple, had not continued to preach about Christ (Acts 5:42)? Or if Isaac Jogues, after being horribly tortured by the Iroquois and making a miraculous escape, had not risked his life all over again by returning to his beloved Indians?

St. Paul, arguably the greatest of all evangelists, is my favorite example, next to Jesus, of a person who was tirelessly persistent. He was beaten with rods and scourged five times with "forty lashes minus one." Once, he was shipwrecked and spent a night and a day in the water. He walked incredible distances and was exposed to all manner of danger. At Lystra, after being dragged to the outskirts of town, stoned, and left for dead, he picked himself up, went back to confront his persecutors (!), and it was there that he converted Timothy, one of his most faithful disciples. In Philippi, where he was publicly flogged, he won over the jailer, along with his entire household. With Paul, as with others in our catalogue of heroes, the greater the suffering, the better the results. The sheer doggedness of the man must have given his followers immense delight. But over and above his unwillingness to give up or give in, he is unforgettable because we see in him a man who positively exults in his suffering (Col. 1:24) and views his trials as so many decorations on the chest of a war hero (2 Cor. 11), a divine boast. Writing from prison, he invites us to imitate him: "Rejoice in the Lord always! I say it again: rejoice!" (Phil. 4:4 NAB). We can do no less.

MEDITATION 7

◆ ◆ ◆ ◆ ◆ ◆

THE GUIDING HAND

THE GUIDING HAND

✦ ✦ ✦ ✦ ✦ ✦

God's guiding hand is everywhere as He weaves His designs into the fabric of everyday life. However, those who are spiritually short sighted see only the underside of a magnificent tapestry. St. Ignatius, the founder of the Jesuit Order, and Walter Scott, the greatest of all Scottish novelists, both wanted to be soldiers when they were young until accidents made them lame. Neither were pleased at the time, but God had other ideas in mind.

Harriet Beecher Stowe was sad when she had to leave her native Connecticut and move to Cincinnati. Her husband, on a meager salary, felt he could serve his wife and children better by accepting a teaching post in the Midwest. And so the family packed up and left behind all that was familiar. The experience was wrenching, and no one felt it more than Mrs. Stowe. Yet Cincinnati inspired her to write *Uncle Tom's Cabin*, the most widely acclaimed novel ever to flow from the pen of an American, for while there, her home became a station on the Underground Railroad for escaped slaves.

Louisa May Alcott, a contemporary of Stowe and the author of *Little Women,* began her career as a nurse, and like Stowe she bowed to circumstances beyond her control. But the same illness that forced her to retire from the medical field afforded her time to write, and it was not long before *Hospital Sketches*, based on real life, catapulted her to literary fame.

God is in charge. He guides and inspires. He also regulates the level of pain. How else does one explain the fact that so many Old and New Testament martyrs were able to bear up under unimaginable torment? Daniel and his companions under Nebuchadnezzar emerged unscathed from the lions' den and white-hot furnace, while in Roman times John the Evangelist withstood boiling oil, St. Polycarp would not burn, and half-starved beasts refused to touch the body of St. Blandina.

In recent times, we have seen the case of a man drowning in freezing water rescued by a bystander so pumped up with adrenaline that he hardly felt the cold. Another person was mauled by a shark so badly that his head alone required thirty stitches. Later, this same man testified to being so numb with shock during the initial seaside attack that he did not experience the slightest pain until after surgery.

Sometimes in life we feel as if we are sleepwalking. Call it unreal, if you will. But God is always at work, with every stroke of the divine chisel carefully measured to produce good, rather than evil. Prison has little to recommend it, and exile is hardly the place where anyone wants to be. Still, literary work of the highest caliber—from a full-length classic such as *Pilgrim's Progress* to O. Henry's marvelous short stories—has been crafted from the confines of a dungeon. Dante wrote the *Divine Comedy* after being forced out of Florence.

One can go further. Persecution of the Faith is, without doubt, an enormity. Many who are innocent suffer intensely. Yet almost invariably, the long-range results are good. Persecution has occurred in virtually all countries, including those that call themselves Catholic, and in every case, religion has emerged stronger. Faith seems to thrive on adversity.

Ethiopia during the 1980s was run by Marxists who hated Christianity. One of the groups slated for extinction was the Mennonite Church, and Mennonite records tell an amazing story. Prior to the persecution, there were fourteen congregations with 5,000 members in all. But when the torture and killing came to an end, the number of congregations had risen to fifty-three with a combined membership of 50,000—a tenfold increase.

What the early Christian Church had to endure is unimaginable. There has never been anything quite like the horror inflicted by a handful of Roman emperors on the followers of Jesus. Still, Christianity triumphed, and to a degree unparalleled in the centuries since. Well could Tertullian say that "the blood of martyrs is the seed of the Church."[8] He knew whereof he spoke, having witnessed the martyrdom of his own father.

So useful has persecution been to the cause of religion that spiritual leaders have actually prayed for it as a means of furthering their cause, and we have already seen a number of examples. St. Ignatius of Loyola hoped that the Jesuits would "never for long remain unharassed by the enmity of the world." Unlike his namesake, Ignatius of Antioch, who asked God for martyrdom and received it, the founder of the Jesuits was content with the world's hatred. He never petitioned the Lord for illness, death, or martyrdom, as did fellow Jesuits Aloysius Gonzaga and John Regis, both of whom have been canonized, but one may be sure that if there had been anything to gain from personal sacrifice of any kind whatever, Ignatius would have been the first to oblige.

How many of us are brave enough to ask God for the heaviest cross He is willing to send? Not many, to be sure. But what each and every one of us *can* do is uncork a bottle of champagne after an untimely setback or an undeserved rebuke. From time to time, it is important to reaffirm one's belief in Divine Providence.

Moments before Christ began to sweat blood in the Garden of Gethsemane, He was at the Last Supper. And what was He doing but *giving thanks* to His heavenly Father (Mt. 26:27). Next to His poignant prayer from the Cross, "Father, forgive them; for they know not what they do" (Lk. 23:34), nothing more startling ever came from the lips of the Savior. And when the two utterances are placed side by side, we have the sum of what it means to be Christian.

Additional insight into the meaning of suffering is contained in Jesus' explanation for why a certain man was born blind: "It was not that this man sinned, or his parents, but that the works of God might be made manifest in him" (Jn. 9:3). And how could they be made manifest if not by cheerful acceptance of the handicap? It is interesting, in this same connection, to note how Our Lord responded when tempted by the devil to work a stupendous miracle for nonbelievers (Mt. 4:6). All would realize who He was, and His life would be spared. But Jesus refused to be drawn: "You shall not tempt the Lord your God" (Mt. 4:7). He had chosen to suffer and to die in order to show His love for the Father and all mankind. Never would He overwhelm those bent on resistance. Never would He coerce the one whose lifestyle precluded an honest search for truth. In short, there would be no diminution of man's noblest faculty: freedom of the will.

The reason, perhaps, why Catholicism has so much to say on the subject of suffering is because the price it has paid for discipleship is greater than that of any other Christian community. It holds no monopoly on martyrdom. Nevertheless, the persecution it has endured from one end of the globe to the other is without parallel, and the penitential practices of its saints are equally remarkable. But this is an aside.

Two final types of pain are worth considering since they affect all of us on a daily basis. Limitation, the first of these, begins at birth. A newborn child is limited in the sense of being utterly dependent. Yet even when childhood gives way to adulthood, there is much to be desired. No one has everything. The world's premier chess player does not win track medals. A college professor may be gifted with ideas, powers of analysis, and rhetorical ability, but he is not likely to be a financial whiz. Beethoven knew no peer in the realm of pianistic virtuosity. His fingers ran up and down the keyboard at mesmerizing speed. But as a boy, he had trouble with math. Deprivation, another word for limitation, is a given this side of heaven.

Sin, as a source of pain, comes second after deprivation since it is not generally thought to exist before the age of reason. It conjures up images of syphilis, AIDS, loss of hair, sclerosis of the liver, obesity, schizophrenia, unemployment, and depression. But worse than physical affliction is a troubled conscience. Guilt can cause hardened criminals to give themselves up long after they have outsmarted the police. Some unburden themselves to casual passersby, while others boast of their cleverness. Still others drive erratically and are picked up for speeding. In the world of fiction, Shakespeare's Lady Macbeth is constantly washing her hands while Raskolnikov, the villain of Dostoevsky's *Crime and Punishment*, marches off to the local constabulary to turn himself in for murder.

Remorse is, of course, healthy as long as it does not result in suicide. Soul tissue behaves like body tissue, and pain is a sign of life. But the answer in Christian terms is neither a washbasin nor a constable. Rather, it is the Sacrament of Reconciliation. "Though your sins are like scarlet, they shall be as white as snow" (Is. 1:18). The door of the confessional is always open, and when we avail ourselves of the grace of penance and come away with a firm purpose of amendment, we feel wondrously light. Praise the Lord!

There is a good deal more to be said on the subject of suffering. But in concluding this, the last of our meditations on the gift of pain, we come, full circle, to the benefits of a religious disposition, and no one makes more sense in this regard than Cardinal Newman, who drank deeply of the cup of suffering and wrote about it[9] as follows:

The Mission of My Life

God has created me to do Him some definite service. He has committed some work to me which He has not committed to another.

I have my mission—I never may know it in this life, but I shall be told it in the next. . . .

I am a link in a chain, a bond of connection between persons.

He has not created me for naught.

I shall do good, I shall do His work,

I shall be an angel of peace, a preacher of truth in my own place while not intending it—if I do but keep His commandments. . . .

Therefore, I will trust Him—whatever, wherever I am.

I can never be thrown away.

If I am in sickness, my sickness may serve Him . . .

If I am in sorrow, my sorrow may serve Him. . . .

He does nothing in vain. . . . He knows what He is about.

He may take away my friends, He may throw me
among strangers;

He may make me feel desolate, make my spirits
sink, hide my future from me—

Still, He knows what He is about.

NOTES

❖ ❖ ❖ ❖ ❖ ❖

1 C.S. Lewis, *The Problem of Pain* (San Francisco: HarperOne, 2001), 93.

2 St. Rose of Lima, *Ad medicum Castillo*, ed. L. Getino (Madrid: La Patrona de America, 1928), 54–55.

3 Rev. Francois Jamart, OCD, *Complete Spiritual Doctrine of St. Therese Lisieux* (New York: Alba House, 1961), 168.

4 Kim Hardey, "From Death to New Life," in *Amazing Grace for Those Who Suffer* (West Chester, PA: Ascension Press, 2002), 165.

5 Brian Caulfield, "A Small Soul for the Lord," *The Latin Mass*, Spring 1999, 72–4, available from http://www.riverbendds.org/index.htm?page=feb00.html.

6 François-René Chateaubriand (vicomte de), *The Memoirs of Chateaubriand*, trans. Robert Baldick (Harmondsworth: Penguin Books in association with Hamish Hamilton, 1965, c1961).

7 Raymond Arroyo, *Mother Angelica: The Remarkable Story of a Nun, Her Nerve, and a Network of Miracles* (New York: Doubleday, 2005), 251.

8 Tertullian, *Apologeticus*, chapter 50.

9 John Henry Newman, "Hope in God—Creator," in *Meditations and Devotions of the Late Cardinal Newman*, ed. W.P. Neville (New York: Longmans, Green, & Co., 1907), 400–401.